N/A

"This is a succinct and highly readable guide that has something for everyone with a sleep problem or question."

— Alfred Lewy, Professor Emeritus of Psychiatry, Oregon Health & Science University

"Make an investment in one of the most important things you can do for your health and happiness: get a good night's sleep. Dr. Johnson-Quijada's engaging book will show you why this is necessary and how to get the most out of sleep."

— Paul J. Zak, PhD. Author of *The Moral Molecule: The Source of Love and Prosperity*

"A delightful, quick read which gets to the heart of how to get a good night's sleep."

— Dinah Miller, M.D. Johns Hopkins University, Department of Psychiatry and Behavioral Sciences, Coauthor of *Shrink Rap: Three Psychiatrists Explain Their Work*

Sleep Well

A "Friend to Yourself" Resource

By Sana Johnson-Quijada, MD

ISBN-13: 978-1530895694
Third Edition

ISBN-10: 1530895693

For more information about this book, visit
http://friendtoyourself.com

Names, situations, and stories herein are the product of the author's imagination. Any resemblance to actual persons, living or deceased, is wholly coincidental.

Contents

Chapter 1

The Hole in Our Self Care

Do you remember the story of Achilles, the Greek hero of the Trojan War? According to legend, when he was a child, his mother held him by the back of his ankles and secretly dunked him in the Styx River, thinking it would make him immortal. And it worked—well, mostly. The magical properties of the water made him invincible, except for the tiny section of skin that did not touch the water, where his mother's fingers gripped him.

Years later, the overachieving and overconfident Achilles was finally brought down in battle when a single arrow pierced his heel, his only vulnerability.

Sometimes, a person's greatest asset becomes their greatest risk. In the case of Achilles, his asset of strength and resilience became the arrogance that left his humble heel exposed to the arrow's mark.

For many of us, sleep has become our Achilles heel.

1

We believe our strength comes from our actions, from our awake selves. If we can control our conscious selves, our awake selves, then everything will be fine. But often our weakness comes from our unconscious, our sleeping selves. Decreasing or weakening our rest can bring us down, perhaps as if struck by an arrow.

For those of you who know me, either through my blog (http://friendtoyourself.com/) or my psychiatric practice, you know that I am a passionate advocate for "being a friend to yourself." Many people also refer to this idea as "self care," the idea that we are not fully useful to anyone else if we are not taking the time to identify and meet our own unique needs.

Being a friend to yourself is more than getting a manicure every now and then, or taking the time to go shopping or watch movies, or doing what seems "fun." In fact, being a friend to yourself often means not doing what you want to do.

That is because being a friend to yourself means taking accountability for yourself—your own happiness, your own health, your own spirituality, and your own connections to the outside world. It means acknowledging that you are not a victim, even though you may have been victimized, hurt, misused, or forgotten.

It means acknowledging that"everything starts and ends with Me."

For most of us, learning to be friends to ourselves is the hardest work we ever do.

Sometimes, being a friend to yourself might feel like you are turning your back on the people who need you, or like you're being selfish, sacrilegious, or even "unfriendly." We live in a world that rewards those who work long hours and who meet everyone else's needs, and celebrates those who are constantly "on" for everyone else. We value doing, doing, doing. Yet when we are carefully tending to our own needs, our own selves—and this begins with sleeping— we don't seem to be doing. We are rarely noticed or thanked when we are taking care of our own needs. Sounds great, right? I can already hear you asking, "Where do I sign up?"

Sarcasm aside, though, think about it.

Pull out your wallet and look at how much money you have inside. How far will that take you? Would it support you through the rest of today? Would it support you for a week? A month? How about the rest of your life? Probably not. You'll need to re-fill your wallet regularly in order for it to sustain you.

How are you keeping it full? How do you get the currency you need to put food on the table and a roof over your head? How do you add what you want to splurge on the ones you love and share with others? It doesn't just magically appear. You have to be intentional about restocking yourself.

Now imagine that the wallet represents a person, in this example, a woman. And what is inside her body are the physical, emotional, and spiritual assets that support her. Her currency is her energy, her positive emotions, her focus, and her motivation, as well as her physical strength, her senses, and even her humor.

How does she spend those assets? If she's like many people I meet, she gives most of them to her children. She's up with the babies (and sometimes the teenagers) in the night. She skips exercising for years on end. It's too hard, she tells herself, when her body is either pregnant or recovering from pregnancy. And she's always so tired, but she never gets to rest.

After seven years of carrying too much leftover baby weight around, she's fed up with it, but her body won't cooperate. She eats whatever food her kids demand, or whatever's handy while she drives them here and there. She's too tired to care that she and her husband haven't had sex in four months, but it does bother her that he looks at so much porn. She can't bring herself to talk to him about it. All she can do at the end of the day is numbly lie in bed and stare at the TV.

Her cell phone is full of phone numbers of other parents from her kids' schools, but she doesn't really know anything about them. She doesn't have time, or energy, to spend on anyone else.

Her middle child has eczema, and is in a nervous stage where he's clingy, cries a lot, and wakes her up in the night to complain about stomachaches. She doesn't want to admit it, but she cannot remember the last time she enjoyed being with him—or any of her kids, for that matter. She loves them, of course. That's what all these long years of sacrifice are about. She just wishes they all treated her better. She snaps at them when they don't appreciate her, yet the kids are her life. She can't imagine a time when they move out, which is something else that keeps her awake at night. She can't remember who she was without them. She'll have to move with them, husband or no husband. What else does she have?

In case it's not obvious, this woman's not very happy. She's not a friend to herself, and if we're honest, she's probably not that nice to anyone else, either. If we're really honest, we'll notice that this woman's family probably enjoys her about as much as she enjoys herself. No one appreciates someone who's too tired to engage, or who acts like a martyr.

This woman's personal wallet has been empty for a long time, and everyone around her is suffering the consequences.

We know that cash doesn't just magically appear in our wallets unless we do something to put it there. So why do we keep waiting for our personal assets to replenish themselves? And why do we keep thinking that staying awake is more valuable, and will get us what we want, to the point of neglecting our own health and self?

It's up to us to each fill our own wallets by taking care of ourselves and taking responsibility for our own assets.

I can go on, but I think you get it. You cannot give what you do not have.

Being a friend to yourself means caring for your body as well as your soul, and understanding that meeting—or ignoring—basic physical needs can lead to complex outcomes. Your exercise, your diet, your water, and yes, especially your sleep, are all worth fighting for.

Now imagine what would happen if that woman took care of her basic needs. Picture her life if she made it a priority to hit the gym a few days a week, even when her kids tugged on her sweatpants and her bathroom floor did not get cleaned. She might have lost that extra twenty pounds by now, and although she would have to keep working and using some of her assets to keep it off, she'll hardly believe how fantastic it feels to live without all that weight.

Picture what her asset levels would be if she did not get up or stay up in the night for her kids every time, but sometimes let them cry it out or get themselves to bed. Imagine if she made her own sleep a priority, and instead of that late-night TV she turned off the lights earlier and went to sleep—or rolled over to connect physically with her husband.

Maybe, on the surface, it would seem like she was opening her wallet less often and not sacrificing as much for her family. She might even seem selfish. But now, when this woman looks in her wallet, there's something there. And when she sees her kids, she not only loves them, but she has the emotional resources to like them. Sometimes they'll even take her breath away.

When we make ourselves a priority, we may appear to give less, but we actually have more for those we love. Just like any bank, we must deposit more than we withdraw if we're going to protect our basic assets. And our bodies are the most important, irreplaceable assets that we've been given.

The choice of how to spend what we have is our own. We are free to choose self care, or not. But when we choose to be friends to ourselves, we don't need a mother or a police officer or the government to strong-arm us to do what's best, because we want to take care of ourselves. That's what being a friend to yourself is all about. And it all starts with sleep.

Questions:

1. What's in your emotional wallet? Take an honest look at your supply of energy, of patience, of love, of strength. How far will it get you?

2. Where are you spending your personal resources?

3. What are you doing to replenish your emotional and physical energy supply?

Chapter 2

Understanding the Physiology of Our Sleep

Of all the ways that we can be friends to ourselves, sleep often gets the least respect. After all, others can see you dieting, exercising, and building relationships. Doctors are there to support you if you need medication. But sleep is a very solitary, and very personal, action.

Maybe that's why sleep has such a bad reputation. We all know how hard it is to function well if we don't get enough sleep. Yet the people I talk to, even when they're physically exhausted and emotionally drained, often describe their need for sleep as a personal weakness. Taking time to refresh themselves, they say, is so much less important than the many things that keep them awake. Sleeping, they tell me, in actions if not in words, is selfish.

Twang. I hear that arrow that pierced Achilles' heel.

9

Sleep may be a solitary activity, happening well outside everyone's sight, but that doesn't mean that it's some kind of mystery. If you are having trouble sleeping, chances are that there's a reason, and a solution.

What is sleep?

To begin, we need to understand what sleep is, why it's important, and how we as humans approach it.

Sleep is a physiologic state, and countless research studies show that it is necessary for both physical and emotional well-being. Sleep has been extensively studied for centuries, and its architecture is well described. Contemporary scientists use a technique called polysomnography, which uses electrodes on a person's scalp to measure their electrical brain activity while they sleep. This allows us to identify patterns in how a person experiences sleep, and to understand their healthy and unhealthy sleep patterns.

When a person is asleep, they experience one of two distinct states—non-REM sleep and REM sleep. Non-REM sleep has four stages, in addition to REM. A person cycles through each stage during the night in periods of approximately ninety minutes.

Sleep Stages	Clinical Features, Normal and Abnormal
Awake	Awake, alert, calm, eyes closed
Stage 1	Drifting in and out of sleep Hypnic myoclonia may occur, causing a sudden jerk that feels like a startle response
Stage 2	Eye movements stop Sleep-panic attacks happen at this stage
Stage 3	Brain activity slows down

Stage 4	Deep sleep, difficult to awaken Bed-wetting (enuresis), night terrors, and sleepwalking (somnambulism) happen at this stage
REM Sleep	Dreams occur, muscles become paralyzed, increased heart rate and blood pressure Penile erections, nightmares, and REM-panic may occur

Normal sleep architecture can be disrupted by many things, including sleep disorders, medication, and the natural aging process. Most of us, at some point, will experience something that impairs sleep efficiency.

Even though we have "standardized" sleep stages, it doesn't mean that we all sleep the same. Sleep is a biological phenomenon, as unique to each of us as our metabolism. It's important to remember this when you are considering how to be a friend to yourself; just because you observe that another person appears to function optimally with only four hours of sleep doesn't mean that your body will react the same way. Many people—like me—can barely get by with nine hours each night. Those disparities might not seem fair, especially if you're a medical student getting four hours less study time per day as your classmates who need less sleep. But take my word for it—no amount of extra studying makes up for depriving your body of what it needs.

Sleep begins in utero; before we ever take a breath of air, babies in our mothers' wombs experience sleep. Then, as we grow and age, our sleep changes. As adults, we spend at least half of our total sleep time in Stage 2 sleep, twenty percent in REM sleep, and the rest spread among the other stages. Infants, however, spend about half their sleep time in deep REM sleep, and older adults sleep mostly in the lighter stages. This is also helpful to remember as we consider our own sleep patterns and sleep architecture, which can occur differently depending on age and genetic makeup.

In addition to our unique biology and our age, the third thing affecting our sleep is our circadian rhythm. This term refers to our own internal sleep-wake clock, which is largely connected to the cycles of light and darkness where you live.

Bear with me for a few sentences as I explain, because the science here is potentially important to gaining your freedom and being actively kind to yourself.

Your circadian rhythm is regulated by how light acts on your retina. Light sends a message through the optic nerve to the brain's circadian pacemaker, the suprachiasmatic nucleus of the hypothalamus. The hypothalamus, in turn, communicates with the pineal gland to turn off production of the hormone melatonin. Melatonin, which is produced in the pineal gland, normally increases when it gets dark, making people feel sleepy, and then decreases when there is light.

This is why our bodies want to sleep when it's dark, and to be awake when it's light. When we surround ourselves with glowing screens and artificially bright rooms, we affect our circadian rhythms.

The hypothalamus also works with the hypothalamic-pituitary adrenal axis in the endocrine system, alongside the autonomic nervous system, to further synchronize our body's functions associated with our sleep-wake clocks. Our need to sleep affects everything from body temperature, to hormone secretion, to urine production, to changes in blood pressure. When it comes to understanding what's keeping us awake, we may think of these functions less often than we think of our circadian rhythm, but they can each be very important to a good night's rest. For example, some people with sleep-panic, which we'll discuss in a later chapter, wake up with a feeling of urinary urgency, which may be related to a dys-regulation of their sleep-wake clock.

Sleep is a complex state affected by many factors. Disturbed, it has a profound effect on an individual's life. When the body refuses to move into the deeper stages of sleep, we call that insomnia. People who suffer insomnia experience difficulty falling asleep and multiple awakenings. Conservatively, we may say that about thirty percent of humans suffer from insomnia at some point in their lives.

It's time to give sleep the respect, and the attention, it deserves.

Questions:

1. How do you understand your sleep?

2. What is the relationship between sleep and your personal identity/how you understand yourself?

3. What happens to your emotions when you don't get enough sleep? How does it change the ways that you react to the people who are most important to you?

Chapter 3

What's Your Sleep Temperament?

Not so long ago, I met Frank. He was—or had been—a fun-loving, spontaneous guy. He fled from organization of any kind. Just saying the word "organize" made him want to ghost out and play hooky. It wasn't fun when things were predictable.

Not that Frank was irresponsible. Work was the one firm construct in his life, and he was fine with waking up, showering, driving, and working until it was time to drive home. But that was as much routine as he wanted. The rest of his life, he told me, he left deliciously to whim. He ate when he was hungry, refused to make plans until the last minute, and went to bed when he was tired—unless there was something more interesting to do, and then in those cases, he didn't bother to go to bed at all.

And for a long time, this made Frank happy.

Lately however, there was a problem. Frank wasn't having fun anymore. Even when he ignored the decisions of others, the expectations of culture, or the clock, a dark cloud had settled over him.

With impressive awareness of his unhappiness and un-bounded self, Frank made an appointment with me to see if I could help. If help meant medication, then he'd swallow the bitter pill. If it meant making appointments and talking to a professional about his problems, then so be it—at least until he found out what had happened to him. "Not forever," he told me. "But I'll stomach what you give me until I can feel normal again."

Frank was being a friend to himself, while also staying true to his own temperament.

When I work with patients who want to improve their sleep, I consider their biopsychosocial model—which means that I want to understand the intertwining of a person's physical symptoms and chemistry are affected by their thoughts, emotions, and environment. As a psychiatrist, I know that if something's going on with the body, often there's an explanation that involves the mind—and vice versa.

In the brilliant book *Outliers*, author Malcolm Gladwell says "the biggest misconception about success is that we do it solely on our smarts, ambition, hustle, and hard work." A lot of our success, Gladwell says, is based on natural abilities and tendencies that we're born with. So one of the first things I did with Frank was to evaluate his temperament—what you might also call his personality—and how it was affecting his physical symptoms.

No two people are alike, but considering a person's gen-eral temperament, and working within their biological design, can help improve the appropriateness and reli-ability of their treatment. Knowing that Frank was nat-urally an able, spontaneous person who prioritized his fun and freedom over his rest and routines helped me work with him toward the best solution.

The human temperament was broken into categories and described almost one hundred years ago by Carl Jung, and today those descriptions are known as Jung Typology. In the 1960s, a mother-daughter pair of researchers developed a test based on Jung's published types. This test, the Myers-Briggs Type Indicator, asked a series of multiple choice questions to try to measure psychological preferences in how people perceive the world and make decisions.

Although there are cultural biases that may influence the test's outcomes, it's a good starting point for understanding what drives a person like Frank, and his behavior around sleep.

I'm especially drawn to the fourth attitude of the temperament (Judgmental or Perceptive) when it comes to sleep—only in my own unsophisticated way, I think of the attitudes of the temperaments as "The Barners" and "The Grazers."

If you have ever been to a farm, you know that some animals like to wander as far away from the barn as they can. They are the ones that are always stretching their necks past their fences, believing the old cliché—the grass really is better over there. They get pleasure from exploration, movement, and trying new things. They like the process of creating options. These are The Grazers. On the other hand, there are animals that appreciate the security of their feed troughs and hay-filled corners. They know their space and understand, deeply and intimately, the routine of the barn. They are comfortable within the fluid mental and physical space, where they can focus their energy and passion on whatever they choose to start and complete. These are The Barners, and they move from decision to decision with the same grace as those Grazers who move from option to option. They are almost like the same T-shirt, inside out.

The flow of moving from completion to completion brings Barners real pleasure, while the flow of creating options and staying inside a process brings Grazers their pleasure.

Both are beautiful designs in their own rights.

One is not better, or safer, than another. But both have inherent weaknesses. Grazers who do not want to get in the barn may find themselves trapped in the jaws of a stronger, faster wolf. Barn animals, on the other hand, face the dangers of what too many boundaries and walls may bring. There are risks either way.

Frank, of course, was a Grazer. When it comes to sleep, Grazers tend to enjoy the late hours. Frank certainly did. "If I plan my play, it loses spontaneity, and then it is not play anymore. I don't get any time to play if I do not stay up, and that's not good for me."

Frank resented any restrictions on his life or schedule that he felt were artificially imposed. His struggle with sleep was one of the consequences of that. He hadn't connected it yet, though. He was charging forward like Achilles, depending on his strengths to guide him.

You do not have to be a Grazer to think this emphasis on play and fun sounds delightful. But here's the thing: if we do not sleep well enough (deep sleep) and long enough (sleep hours), over time, we lose the ability to physically heal our bodies and our minds enough to enjoy our play.

If a Grazer's kids don't get to sleep until nine o'clock, and Mr. Grazer thinks he needs three hours to "wind down," then he's going to bed at midnight. If he has to get up for work at five, that leaves him very little space to heal, to lay down memories, to restore his neurochemistry, or to deal with inflammation in his body and mind.

Our brains change over time. We cannot replenish our hormones and neurotransmitters, and that makes us more vulnerable to mental and physical illnesses. It decreases our ability to respond to psychotropic medication. Genes that were dormant awaken, and new onset diseases demonstrate themselves.

Frank had some fantastic, creative aspects to his temperament, but choosing to use them in a way that would protect his biology was his sleep-salvation. He didn't resent it when it was his choice. He didn't feel trapped.

Doing what is natural for our temperaments makes it possible to achieve our best through the path of least resistance. Rather than forcing change that seems like nothing but effort, drudgery, and dragging feet, time loses some of its heaviness as we get caught up in inner and outer congruence. To make this specific to our sleep needs, we can use our temperaments to serve us rather than against us if we pair what is natural with our sleep needs.

Questions:

1. How does your temperament play into your sleep habits?

2. How could you use your temperament to better your treatment of yourself, how you befriend yourself through sleep?

3. How much are you really sleeping? Keep a sleep journal (on the next page) for a week and see how it looks.

4. After a week, review your sleep journal with your physician. Together, decide if you are having difficulty with sleep initiation (falling asleep), staying asleep (sleep maintenance), and/or falling back to sleep. Discuss treatments and options specific for your needs.

Sleep Journal

Date begun: _____   Date ended: _____

	Day 1	Day 2	Day 3	Day 4	Day 5	Day 6	Day 7	Average
Bedtime (the previous night)								
Wake time								
Total sleep time (hours)								
Number of awakenings during the night								

Caffeinated drinks (number) ● Before noon							
● Between 12pm-6pm							
● After 6pm							
Exercise (number of minutes)							
Naps (number of minutes)							

Chapter 4

Sleep Hygiene

When Frank came in to see me, he said he had lost himself. He felt like his personality had changed. Frank knew he was suffering, but not why. He was only able to identify that he wasn't himself, and he could not sleep well anymore.

This is often a scary place for patients to be. It is a great unknown. "It could be anything." They fear some dramatic disease. They often also fear coming to a psychiatrist.

Who knows what a psychiatrist will do to them?

Ahem.

Using the biopsychosocial model, I was able to see more of what was happening with Frank. We did tests and sent them to the lab, got him in to see his primary doctor for a physical, and talked about possible "life-stressors," as well as his personal support structure. He kept a sleep journal, and we started medication.

Not surprisingly, none of this was as hard for spontaneity-loving, routine-averted Frank as were the sleep hygiene rules I insisted he follow.

Sleep hygiene refers to the habitual behaviors, or "grooming," we do to take care of our sleep.

I almost lost Frank there. He didn't object to having his veins poked and his mind prodded, but telling him to set rules for sleep was challenging his culture. Even in his lowest state, Frank had enough juice to know that he was a night owl, and he had a hard time redefining himself as something else. It exhausted him just to think about it.

We weren't talking about changing Frank's temperament. That would be impossible. We were talking about his home culture.

His temperament had run up against his treatment, and we needed to try a different approach.

I pulled out his sleep journal. Frank turned his body away and looked at me sideways. He could feel me trying to box him in with data. Instead, I told him I wanted him get the information so he could decide what he wanted to do.

I gave him the information, and we set a deadline for his own research. If he did the work and disagreed with my conclusions, we would find another way forward. If he did not do the work on time—which was a real possibility given his lack of energy and focus (who among us can focus when we don't sleep well?)—Frank would agree to treatment based on my recommendations until his brain illness improved sufficiently to allow him to do more for himself.

These were the Sleep Hygiene Rules I gave Frank, and that I now give to you.

As you read them, keep in mind that these are less about rules and regulations and more about personal culture and home culture. Keep on!

Sleep Hygiene, according to Dr. Q

1. **The bedroom is only for sleep and for sex.** This means no food, no phone, and no TV. If you are not having sex, then all you get to do here is sleep. This might be an adjustment for the entire family, especially if your partner is used to clicking on the late news or the kids want you to read them stories in your bed. But your subconscious has to recognize this bedroom place as a sanctuary, and not the place to read one last chapter or check Twitter. (I have yet to have someone tell me that this rule improved their sex life, but one would think...)

2. **No daytime naps longer than twenty minutes.** If you are tired and have the luxury of lying down during the daytime, do it! But set your alarm to wake you up in twenty minutes, and then make sure you wake up fully. You can take these "power naps" twenty times a day if you want to, as long as they are no more than twenty minutes at a time. Anything longer will reduce your homeostatic drive, which is your perceived need to sleep when it is bedtime.

3. **Exercise, but not before bed.** Exercise during the day can help to regulate your sleep cycle by making your body tired at night, but make sure you do not crowd it against sleep initiation. Try to get 40-60 minutes of aerobic exercise, 5-7 days a week. Look at it like a pill, prescribed by a doctor. This is something you need to do not necessarily for your waistline, but for your medical and emotional health. Every day, tell yourself, "I'm exercising so

that I will feel good, so that I will sleep well, and so that I can do what I want in life." Some of my patients tell me, "I'm exercising for my brain!"

4. **Keep the lights dim before bed, and turn off the screens early.** As we saw in Chapter Two, darkness releases melatonin from the pineal gland in our brains, which helps to regulate our sleep cycle. Light suppresses it. Melatonin is a cornerstone in sleep architecture. Keeping your face six inches from the computer or TV before you lie down doesn't give your body much time to turn itself off. (Some people who feel they must be on the computer or TV before bed have found that wearing sunglasses for at least the last thirty minutes helps.)

5. **Go to bed and get out of bed at the same time every day.** Enough said there.

6. **If you go to bed but cannot fall asleep in thirty minutes, get up and do something else until you feel sleepy.** Then go to bed and try again. Refer back to the other rules when choosing your activities (no screens, no reading in bed, etc.).

7. **No caffeine in the second half of your day.** Period. No matter how good that iced latte looks, decaffeinated is the way to go!

8. **Do not use alcohol to sleep.** Alcohol is a depressant of your central nervous system's chemical messengers and also blocks deep sleep by targeting the GABA receptors. Alcohol also relaxes your airway, increasing your risk of obstructive sleep apnea and decreasing oxygen to the brain and body.

9. **Do not smoke before bed or if you awaken from sleep.** Nicotine is stimulating. (By the way, it also decreases blood flow to the penis, complicating the other permissible bedroom activity...)

10. **If you cannot fall asleep in thirty minutes, consider taking a sleep aid.** Do not take any over-the-counter sleep aids except melatonin, valerian root, or chamomile. Other over-the-counter sleep aids almost all contain diphenhydramine, which actually blocks your deep sleep. You may end up sleeping a longer amount of time, but you will not be getting restorative sleep. If you talk to a doctor about a prescription sleep aid, avoid benzodiazepines. Benzodiazepines, such as diazepam (Valium), temazepam (Restoril), clonazepam (Klonopin), alprazolam (Xanax), or lorazepam (Ativan), target GABAergic neurons, the same receptors alcohol hits, which also block deep sleep. It's like taking alcohol in a pill.

Prescription sleep aids that don't block deep sleep or disrupt sleep architecture include atypical benzodiazepine receptor ligands such as zolpidem (Ambien), eszopiclone (Lunesta), or zaleplon (Sonata). Trazodone (Desyrel) is also safe for sleep structure and maintenance. The newest sleep aid that I would consider a Friend to Yourself resource is Belsomra.

Sometimes people will find that combining sleep aids, such as taking a small piece of zolpidem with a small piece of trazodone with melatonin, is more effective than using only one agent by itself; they target more paradigms of healing. Some medications wash quickly out of the body, and some last the full night, so you can fall asleep quickly, stay asleep, and not awaken with a hangover.

11. **Do not sleep with your pets or children.** It is not personal. It is sleep hygiene. Pets and children are disruptive, and no one gets the rest they need. Get the sweet buddy-dog out of bed.

Questions:

1. Consider the list of sleep hygiene tools. What will be the hardest of these for you to implement? Which do you want to skip? Why do you want to skip those aspects of sleep hygiene? Is it something to do with your home culture? Habits?

2. If you're having trouble sleeping, try implementing as many of the sleep hygiene tools as you can for at least a week. Then look. Has your sleep changed?

3. If you can't implement all the "rules" of sleep hygiene, why not give yourself the pick of the "chocolate box?" Try a few. Take what you want. Taste. Think. Rethink. Try out a few more. Give your family and yourself a chance to accommodate changes. These sleep habits are here to serve you, not you to serve them.

Chapter 5

Anxiety and Its Unnerving Effect on Sleep

The more I talked to Frank, the more I could see a clear picture.

Anxiety bubbled, frothed and infused the air when Frank's wife, Yesenia, accompanied him to a session. Yesenia could barely catch her breath. She was not in treatment with me. Her husband was. Yet it was Yesenia who filled our space.

There was barely room for Frank and I to speak, or to sit quietly, with all that anxiety around. Frank was breathing faster every moment, and his face didn't have much color.

Where to start?

It was too early in our work together to expect Frank to know this, but emotions are contagious. Anxiety is very contagious. Even when it's not our own, anxiety influences how our genes express themselves. So my patient wasn't only Frank. My patient included the system he lived in: his home life, his wife, his kids, his work, and so forth.

Especially his wife. Because of Yesenia's untreated emotional disease, Frank's emotional disease worsened. The inverse would be true, as well. Health begets health. We go round and round, gaining momentum, like a big ball of hard-packed snow gathering speed and girth as it rolls down the mountain.

Anxiety grows. Where to start?

For many people who are experiencing temporary or situational sleep issues, addressing hygiene is enough. However, for some the problems come from a deeper source. Some people have difficulty falling asleep or staying asleep because of illness.

Understanding that our behaviors can be related to illnesses and conditions can be uncomfortable. It takes a lot of courage to recognize that medical illness has a relationship to how we feel and behave. It can challenge our very identity, how we define ourselves. "Who am I?" feels different.

We can't sleep.

No one is quite as mean to "Me" than we are to ourselves.

However, no one else has the same opportunity to be an advocate for "Me," either. Even a friend.

Since our brains are connected to the rest of our bodies, and emotions and behaviors come from the brain, we can make a truce. Because even though our very biology is victimizing us, so to speak, we don't have to be the victim. We are free to choose.

By acknowledging and addressing the root of an issue, by choosing to advocate for ourselves, we move past the place of being a victim.

The good news is that most medical and psychological-based sleep problems can be recognized, diagnosed, and treated. Things will get better, and you will find yourself again. And you can begin with something as seemingly simple as sleep.

If you've implemented all of the sleep hygiene steps recommended in the previous chapter and still have not found relief, consider whether your body is showing any of the symptoms of a medical or biological condition. A medical professional is able to diagnose the underlying issues for your specific sleep problems. Be a friend to yourself and seek the personalized attention you need.

There are a number of medical and psychological issues that can make it hard to get the rest our bodies need.

There are a number of medical illnesses that can affect sleep health, but in this little book, we will look specifically at anxiety in this chapter, and sleep apnea in the next.

When I was a just a girl with dirty feet and pigtails, spending the summer on my grandparents' farm with my three similarly dirty big brothers, we took Grandpa's two John Deere tractors out for a drive. We delighted in the enormous strength in those beasts, the tires taller than me.

I rode with one brother, following the other two up ahead. We raced across the pasture. The boys were yelling at each other, provoking and jocular. I was, as usual, amazed at my luck to have the boys for my own.

Somewhere before we lost interest and after we lost sense, the first tractor hit mud. My brother and I, still behind them, hollered with laughter. We jeered as those monster tires dug deeper and deeper. Oh, the tears of delight...right up until we followed them into our own mud-sink.

All I remember about that field is how wet the ground was beneath the tall grass. The green came up almost to the middle of the tractors, and the blades were wide and thick. We got to business, pulling grass and feeding it under the muddy tires, thinking to build traction. An hour later, the sharp blades of grass had taught our hands a lesson and the tractors still wouldn't move. We tramped back to the barn to confess to Grandpa.

I remember that grass when I'm faced with patients or friends suffering with anxiety. I feel like I am once again pulling grass, feeding it under spinning wheels, hoping that it will help them move again.

Anxious conditions feel like Grandpa's John Deere, stuck in the mud with spinning wheels. We behave ineffectively. Our own inner dialogue sounds like it's coming from a stranger. We feel differently toward the world around us, toward the people who once were the reason we made those choices, and toward the work that once mattered.

Panic

I had a favorite mentor, an attending doctor in my medical school rotation, once tell me, "Anxiety is what makes us work hard. If we didn't have anxiety, we'd all be slobs. We'd stink. We wouldn't get our homework done. We wouldn't say as many nice things."

His comments were funny. Until they weren't.

The most extreme form of anxiety at any time of day is panic. Unless you've been through one, no one can grasp the horror of a panic attack. It's a combination of fright, chest pain, ringing in the ears, numbness in the arms and hands, a sense that something horrible is going to happen, and more...and it comes on suddenly, often without warning.

When it comes during sleep, it awakens people who were just the moment before completely blacked out to the world. Suddenly, without provocation, they are fully alert. This usually happens while they are in an earlier stage of sleep, and so the response isn't associated with a dream.

This is what we mean by "sleep-panic."

One panic attack does not mean that a person has, or will develop, a full-blown panic disorder. In fact, about one-third of people who have had panic attacks do not develop a disorder. A diagnosable sleep panic disorder emerges when panic attacks become recurrent and at least one of three things happen:

- *anticipatory anxiety*, in which a person starts worrying constantly about having another panic attack
- the individual worries about the consequences of the anxiety attack (i.e., having a heart attack, going crazy)
- *phobic avoidance*, in which a person starts changing their behaviors related to the panic attacks (i.e. changing their bed partner, place of sleep, or other "causality" inappropriately linked to explaining why they are going through these horrors.)

Panic throws out sticky tendrils to snag any effort to get out of ourselves, to connect with others, to empathize, to hear, touch, see, smell, taste anything outside of "Me." It is distracting and, worse, it is suspicious. The person who was once open to the world around her now doubts the intentions of others, including medical professionals. They are suspicious of the treatments I recommend. They have trouble hearing past the white noise, the static that reminds me of the old analog TVs with antennae that were always out of focus, always blurred with a little static. That's anxiety.

Panic can feel like a heart attack, and many people go to the emergency room repeatedly seeking medical explanations, convinced that there is something "wrong" with their bodies. In fact, anxiety can be caused by a variety of medical problems, which also disrupt sleep. Examples include seizures, inappropriate sleeping medications (like the ones covered in the last chapter), stimulating medications, reflux esophagitis, and alcohol or drug addiction.

People with panic disorder have more insomnia than the general population, but specifically, more middle-of-the-night and early morning awakenings. These awakenings are not necessarily related to sleep-panic attacks, although the majority of people with some kind of panic disorder do experience sleep-panic attacks at some point in their life, although less frequently than daytime panic attacks.

It is suspected that there is also a distinct sleep-panic syndrome, which represents a variant of panic disorder and affects about ten percent of all people with panic disorder. Patients report that sleep-panic is often brought on by feeling tired and sleep deprived. Yet sleep-panic pulls them out of sleep and leaves them with insomnia, unable to drift off again. It can be vicious cycle.

They have found that some people suffer recurrent sleep-panic attacks, even when they do not experience daytime panic attacks. Interestingly, although sleep-panic attacks are just as terrible as daytime panic attacks, individuals with sleep-panic have less social or occupational disability, and fewer phobic limitations like agoraphobia, than do people with a more general panic disorder. However, sleep-panic syndrome is also associated with more depressive disorders and, not surprisingly, insomnia.

This is nothing to take lightly or try to ignore.

A teenager I treat began responding to her medication. Her mom complained that her room was a mess. She was less prompt to obey, and she started voicing her opposing opinions more.

She wasn't serious about complaining, though. Without the anxiety, her true teenage personality was coming through, and her mom was getting to know her for the first time. This was better than anything they had hoped for. The girl wasn't throwing up, having panic attacks, or avoiding every social experience. She was making eye contact, and she was able to speak in class for the first time in years. She tells me she can't even think about how she felt before. It was so bad.

It is really hard for anyone who has never suffered from debilitating anxiety to realize the level of suffering and terror it causes. Someone who may look stuck up, aloof, disinterested, quiet, bored, may in fact be at hell's door.

Generalized Anxiety Disorder

Generalized anxiety disorder, (or GAD) turns us into what we unscientifically call "worrywarts." For at least six months, there are preoccupied thoughts and worries, usually accompanied by discomforts like restlessness or feeling keyed up or on edge, being easily fatigued, difficulty concentrating or the feeling of the mind going blank, irritability, muscle tension, and sleep disturbance.

People with GAD often have difficulty falling asleep because their muscles are tense and their minds won't relax. Although they may not have sleep-panic attacks (although illnesses often do overlap), a person living with general anxiety disorder suffers from a lower sleep quality. It's not as restful.

People who experience generalized anxiety disorder often suffer from *hyperarousal insomnia*. Already "on edge" and worrying constantly about multiple details of their lives, they find themselves unable to sink into a good sleep. Treatment for hyperarousal insomnia includes things that will relax the body and mind, like good sleep hygiene, regular exercise, progressive relaxation exercises, or a hot bath before bed.

Getting through everyday life with something as subtle as GAD can be devastating. Some people try to explain away the consequences as the result of an injustice, a personality quirk, or simply neglect. But it could be different. The same rude, distrustful teacher, or the rejection from a crush, or the quiet mike and the uncomfortable audience – those moments could have been different with better brain health. The same stressors could have been perceived very differently by a healthy brain, and the life-story would have then, in turn, been told differently.

It takes courage to believe that the effect of our negative thoughts and distorted perceptions could indeed have that pervasively profound effect. It takes courage to consider that medical treatment can, likewise, profoundly change our quality of life.

As Nancy A. Payne, of New York University Silver School of Social Work, wrote about treating brain illness, "There is tremendous satisfaction gained from facilitating the transition from profound illness to equally profound recovery."

Another sleep condition related to generalized anxiety disorder is *psychophysiologic insomnia*, an anxiety disorder that develops from behavioral conditioning. In this case, everything about sleep becomes a trigger to a person's anxiety about falling asleep or staying asleep. When they are awake, they feel a lot of anxiety about getting to sleep. If they fall asleep at all, they are often too anxious to fall into a deep sleep, and thus are easily awakened, causing a vicious circle of anxiety and insomnia.

Stress Response Syndrome

Stress response syndrome is a general category that encompasses more familiar names, such as posttraumatic stress and adjustment disorders. These are the result of life-threatening events and trauma.

Sometimes when traumatic events happen, a sudden influx of calcium can flood into the cells in a certain part of the brain, and it actually kills those cells. The result is a medical illness that can threaten the way we see the world around us.

Stress response syndrome affects a person's REM sleep, which is the sleep stage when we experience dreams. A person will jerk awake, showing signs of panic, vividly remembering a horrible dream related to their initial traumatic experience. This is different from sleep-panic, because it happens in a different stage of sleep and is associated with a specific dream recollection.

People with stress response syndrome also are more likely to experience hyperarousal, making it difficult to fall asleep in the first place, leading to initial insomnia.

Obsessive-Compulsive Disorder

Obsessive compulsive disorder, or OCD, is an illness in which we perceive things that at some level we understand are not likely nor true. These fears are called *egodystonic*—we can tell that our fears don't make sense.

For example, my thoughts may be preoccupied with the fear that I just ran over a person with my car. Even though at some level I know I didn't, I might be compelled to drive back and forth for hours, looking for the victim where I fear the accident happened. Even though, if asked outright if any of it made any sense, I'd say no.

Fears consistent with our inner selves are *egosyntonic*. We all have features of this disorder. But some people experience it to the full, terrifying extent. In its diseased states, we see this in disconnected thought form disorders such as schizophrenia.

But back to obsessive-compulsive disorder. It is a chronic disorder that results in disabling obsessions and/or compulsions. Obsessions are uncontrollable, spontaneous, and intrusive thoughts. Compulsions are repetitive, ritualistic behaviors (like checking or hand washing) or mental acts (like counting or repeating words). Obsessions drive the compulsions, leaving a person to feel as if something terrible will happen if they don't perform the ritual.

Obsessive-compulsives generally view their symptoms as ego-dystonic, or against their nature, and they are able to recognize their fears as unrealistic. They don't want to do the compulsions over and over again, but by force of the obsession they cannot help it.

These obsessive thoughts are often terrifying and keep people from sleeping. Even once they fall asleep, the quality of sleep can be poor, because their anxiety doesn't necessarily fall asleep when their bodies do. This has similarities to hyperarousal insomnia.

Parasomnias

Parasomnias are sleep disorders that occur during specific stages of sleep or during the transition from wakefulness to sleep. People may have more than one parasomnia, which may be stress-related or due to irregular sleep schedules or poor sleep hygiene. Many issues occur in children, who often outgrown them. However, some do not, and parasomnias can continue into adulthood.

Sleepwalking is an example of a parasomnia. The sleepwalker gets out of bed while sleeping and walks around (somnambulism). This typically happens in the first third of the night, while the person is in Stage 4 sleep. Like sleep terror disorder, the sleepwalker is unaware and unresponsive to attempts at communication. It is very difficult to awaken a sleepwalker, and the person will not remember sleepwalking.

Alcohol and Drug Disorders

People suffering from anxiety disorders have statistically higher comorbid rates of alcohol problems. Many people who use alcohol like to rationalize that they use it to treat their anxiety symptoms. After all, even Hippocrates once said, "Wine drunk with equal quantity of water puts away anxiety and terror."

Well, that's not necessarily true. Panic and anxiety disorders often stem from alcohol use, rather than helping them. Remember, we heal during deep sleep, anything that blocks deep sleep—like alcohol—in turn blocks healing.

Alcohol has a dramatic effect on sleep. Not only does it disrupt sleep architecture and decrease REM sleep, it also can create a psychological dependence (GABAergic). Alcohol is effective as a sedative, but as tolerance develops the dose must be increased to get the same effect.

When the sleep architecture becomes more impaired, causing fragmented dreams and sleep, the alcohol user subsequently experiences more daytime sleepiness and fatigue.

Other artificial, and potentially detrimental, stimulants include nicotine, illicit drugs (cocaine, amphetamines), caffeine, diet aids, and even decongestants. These can all induce anxiety symptoms, which in turn affect the way that we sleep.

Some prescription medication can cause anxiety symptoms, including stimulants such as Ritalin, cardiovascular medications, steroids, and anticonvulsants. Even anti-anxiety medications, like the GABAergic benzodiazepines we've discussed, can cause anxiety, especially when used incorrectly. Anxiety symptoms can appear as a side effect of taking a medication and also from withdrawal when you stop. Be sure to discuss everything you are taking with your physician, regardless of how benign or unrelated it might seem.

If you think you suffer from sleep-panic or a variation of sleep anxiety, talk to your doctor and schedule a complete medical exam to rule out physical disorders like sleep apnea, which we will discuss in the next chapter. You'll be asked to describe your anxiety symptoms and your sleep, and to identify stressors in your life and your personal and family medical history. Our purpose here is to identify and treat any underlying problems that are causing the sleep-panic or anxiety. In this context, poor sleep is the symptom of a disorder, not the focus of the treatment.

Based on your responses and what your doctor observes, the next steps may be screening tests, which will require a blood sample, and perhaps a sleep study (polysomnogram). If there is indeed an underlying medical disease, your doctor can guide you through the treatment, which should relieve your anxiety symptoms and allow you to experience rest.

If a medical cause is ruled out, your primary care provider may refer you to a psychiatrist to help with a diagnosis and medication management. A psychiatric evaluation is important to rule out anxiety disorders or comorbid psychiatric illnesses. Your sleep disorder may not get better unless the comorbid psychiatric illness is also treated.

Never stop taking medication without consulting your doctor. Because of the effects these medications have on mood and the way they affect anxiety centers in the brain, removing them from your system can leave you in an acute state of anxiety and insomnia. If one medication doesn't work or has side effects, be patient and try others. There are many good medications for anxiety and each person responds uniquely. Also, more medications are being developed all the time and we are fortunate to have many options.

Regular cognitive behavioral therapy and psychotherapy are also important treatment options for sleep-panic and anxiety, especially in combination with medication. There are many different therapy techniques that are helpful in different situations. Examples are relaxation therapy, cognitive behavioral therapy (useful in diminishing anxiety and teaching strategies), and psychotherapy focused on the psychosocial causes of anxiety.

If you think anxiety may be impairing your sleep, discuss it with your doctor. You deserve good sleep. Give yourself the chance to achieve consistent, sound sleep. Be a friend to yourself.

Questions:

1. How have you experienced the contagion of emotions? How have you seen it play out in others?

2. Do you think that there may be more than unhealthy sleep hygiene involved in your sleep problems?

3. What will decrease your barriers to entry into medical care?

4. How are you still free to choose, even if you are being victimized by your own biology?

5. How do you identify yourself, your "Me," even when you can't trust your own biology?

Chapter 6

Obstructive Sleep Apnea

Not long ago, I stood at the edge of the pool and watched as my niece swam, underwater, for the length of the pool. She popped up like an otter – slick, water rolling off her, and smiling like nothing in the world would bother her.

The timer showed her that she beat her record for holding her breath.

My niece would have liked to have added another lap before coming up for air, but at some point, her body wouldn't let her. Humans need to breathe!

Sometimes, the human body does that same holding-the-breath trick while it's sleeping. The medical term for when a person stops breathing for more than ten seconds during sleep is called apnea. When it happens more than thirty times in a night, it is called Obstructive Sleep Apnea (OSA).

Generally speaking, what happens is that the tube through which air goes from your mouth to your lungs, called the pharynx, collapses for a number of seconds, over and over throughout your sleep. You stop breathing, and your body is deprived of oxygen, "anoxia." This is often, though not always, caused by excess body-weight putting pressure on your airways.

The oxygen deprivation affects every cell, organ, system in a person's body because every bit of us needs oxygen to survive. When the brain senses that there isn't enough oxygen arriving with the red blood cells, it sends a message to the heart to pump faster, and to work harder. "Get working! Pump more oxygen-carrying red blood cells!"

The heart dutifully pumps, like a champion.

The heart muscle walls grow thicker, but at the same time the heart muscle itself is not getting enough oxygen. (Nothing in the body is.) At some point the heart walls grow too thick for the limited oxygen to support, and they start to die.

Obstructive Sleep Apnea is a leading cause of early heart attack.

Picture this story; a young father—let's call him Jake—is playing basketball with his buddies from high school on a Sunday. They're joking around, slapping each other's butts (because, help us, that's what they do!). Sweat is rolling down his face. He's heavier after three kids, but he's trying to lose the "baby weight." He snores so loudly that his wife has to wear earplugs. Jake has been playing hard for about thirty minutes. He's running down the court, guarding Tom. Everyone's running, heaving, and breathing hard. Tom makes the shot, and they're all slapping each other's butts again. One of the guys is throwing the ball back into play when someone laughs at Jake. "Hey, Jake! Get up!"

Jake dies. His wife and gorgeous kids are left to live life without his laughter, his counsel, and that noisy snoring his wife would do anything to hear again. Jake's community is man-down.

I wrote this out in what may seem like almost tasteless detail only because this is how it happens. I wish it didn't, and I want it to stop. It is as horrible as you imagine. Obstructive sleep apnea is a deadly sleep disorder.

Additionally, over time, the brain cells change and diseases develop there, secondary to anoxia. Without oxygen, brain cells die, and any variety of brain diseases develop, including early dementia, depression, anxiety, and more.

When we don't get enough oxygen at night, our brains don't get enough restorative sleep, even if we're in bed for hours. We don't feel rested! We're constantly being pulled out of a deeper sleep into a state where our pharyngeal muscles can take over, push open, and allow a breath of precious oxygen. But that requires an awake brain, so all night we "wake up" over and over to breathe. We move from a deep sleep stage to a lighter, more awake stage of sleep over and over throughout the night.

We are then set up for an exhausted struggle throughout the day. Our eyes may be open, but our brains are actually dropping into the early stages of sleep. Daytime sleepiness happens, until boom! You're falling asleep while driving.

You're probably also eating more. Yup. Good news after more good news. Our stimulation-craving brains push us to eat more food than we need, just to release a few more hormones to keep us awake. Eating and food is stimulating for a brief period. But eating more leads to increased weight, and obesity, which then pushes down harder on our poor, suffering airway at night, and Obstructive Sleep Apnea worsens! (It's almost impossible to lose weight while suffering untreated OSA, by the way.)

Now why would the pharynx collapse? Generally it's because the muscles just can't stay open under all that weight. We're too heavy. Those poor oxygen molecules are out of luck spelunking through the narrowing tunnel.

And if this isn't bad enough, the oxygen deprivation associated with sleep apnea makes it more difficult for men to achieve and keep their erections. Bummer!

Most people aren't aware of their own sleep apnea problems, and they aren't fully conscious during the cycles of the night. Often it's the spouse or partner of a patient who first notices the sudden silence and then the panicked gasping that startles the night's peace.

The best way to confirm and get an official OSA diagnosis is through a sleep study, a polysomnogram. While you sleep in a controlled lab environment, specialists will observe your brain activity, as well as your oxygen levels, using an electroencephalogram. The primary treatment for apnea is a machine that pushes air into the airway to keep it open – either a BiPAP or CPAP. While these are life-saving devices, I often meet with some resistance from my patients about wearing them. One patient in particular was young, not obese, and looked healthy. Mark exercised regularly, yet in a sleep study he tested positive for Obstructive Sleep Apnea. He tried wearing a CPAP for a while, but confessed that he stopped because he doesn't feel sexy in it. Actually, his words were that he felt "like I'm wearing a jock-strap on my face." He told me he preferred to snore loudly, go silent, then gasp, over and over, all night.

I don't blame Mark for this response. It is what it is. But I don't think anyone had ever told my patient why he must wear CPAP, or how his brain was screaming for oxygen. He didn't know that this contributed to why his anxiety was not responding to his medications. Why his Cialis wasn't working anymore. Why his ankles were swelling. So we talked about how continuing this severe oxygen deprivation was gifting his wife with a future impotent man. About how every day he enjoyed fewer and fewer functioning brain cells. About how he risked an early death from heart attack.

Just thinking about Mark and Jake's stories makes me take a deep breath and say a prayer of gratitude for the air, oxygen, and life I experience. He did, too, and he agreed to give the CPAP another chance.

CPAP is 99% effective when used. It works. It is not always the easiest treatment to tolerate for many reasons, but it is worth fighting for. You might need to make multiple visits to your primary care practitioner to get that refer-ral to your sleep lab. Or it may take multiple visits to your sleep specialist, trying one sleep mask after another and then another, until you finally find one that keeps a good seal on your face through the night. There are a mountain of barriers, more than Bilbo toward Smaug, that you will trek across, and you'll need as much courage as a hobbit.

If you have, or think you might have, sleep apnea, be a friend to yourself and find out. This is a serious medical condition, but nothing to feel embarrassed and ashamed by. It just is what it is.

You, too, have the chance to feel the sense of accomplish-ment my niece felt when she came up for air. Accepting treatment is that wonderful. We could celebrate. It's all perspective.

Questions:

1. Have you had a sleep study? If not, what are your barriers to getting one?

2. Do you have any recommendations for those of us suffering and ashamed?

3. Why are you compliant with some medical recommendations but not others? Do you distrust the recommendations? Do you think they are "worth it?" Is it coming from temperament? Achilles?

4. How can you use your brilliance and natural talent to protect yourself, in humility, from your natural weaknesses?

Conclusion: The First Step to Being a Friend to Yourself

Like a ghoul that won't die, the confusion over self care versus selfish care comes back to haunt us again and again. People see the word "self" and start to make assumptions. They imagine that a person who focuses on themselves must be toxic to her family and coworkers, only interested in doing what she wants, when she wants it, for as long as she wants. They picture the people who throw their needs into our faces faster than we can turn our heads.

And no one wants to be that person.

But remember, being a friend to yourself is not the same as indulging yourself. Self care is not about doing what you want. It is about giving yourself what you need. Sleep, in this instance, is not a luxury. It is a necessity.

During sleep, we heal from injuries, both physical and mental. These treatments are often better than medicine when it comes to processing and treating stress. When we sleep, we allow our broken neuronal connections to regenerate. We re-stock our pantry with ingredients like cortisol, hormones, and neurotransmitters that help us concoct well-nourished thinking, kind behaviors, and stable emotions. During sleep, our memories find their place in the folds between our cells and root down into our minds.

I have seen regular, restorative sleep bring someone from a place of mental decline to no longer needing psychotropic medication. Everything works better with sleep.

So what is keeping us from it?

Sometimes, sleep will be the thing that you most need to give yourself, while other times you may find that your elf-care structure has other priorities. You are a complex person with many intersecting paradigms, including your general physical health and biology, genetic predispositions, coping skills, what you do to your body, what is done to your body (such as physical trauma), emotional triggers, and spirituality.

We started this "Friend to Yourself" series of booklets with "Sleep" because it's the most commonly overlooked building block to good health. Investing your energies in yourself, and in the world around you, can be more objective when that emotional wallet is well stocked.

So if you're tired during the day, have irregular sleep hours, or are feeling emotional and irritable, start with sleep hygiene. Keep it simple.

When schedule conflicts or temptations seduce us into confusion, or when a project with a seemingly insurmountable deadline looms, or when the siren song of just one more story on Yahoo! News tempts—it's then that we need the commitment to be a friend to ourselves and do what we need, not what we want. When a loved one wants to talk to us, or a conflict grows, or when we mistake good parenting for enabling our children's bad sleeping habits, our friend Me reminds us of the priority of sleep.

Tomorrow, our friend whispers, we can do those things that must be done. Now, it's time to sleep.

If you are exhausted, overwhelmed, struggling to get enough rest to fill your emotional wallet, the choice is yours. Choose to be a friend to yourself. Choose to sleep.

Be a friend to yourself.

Appendix: Drowsy Driving

We've talked about why getting enough sleep is important for your personal health and emotional safety. Without enough sleep, you can't take care of yourself. However, if that's not enough to convince you that sleep matters, I recently read these statistics from the National Institute of Health, which make the case for why addressing your sleep health matters not only for you, but also for the people around you.

Drowsy driving in the United States:

- There are about 100,000 police-reported crashes per year where driver drowsiness is a principal cause.

- About 4 percent of all auto crash fatalities are sleep related.

- At least 71,000 people are injured each year in crashes involving driver drowsiness.

- At least 1 million crashes (about one-sixth of the total) are caused by lapses in driver attention; such lapses are typically associated with lack of sleep.

Who is at risk?

- Drivers who are sleep deprived or fatigued.
- Young drivers. A North Carolina study found that 55 percent of sleep-related crashes involved drivers between the ages of 16 and 25; 78 percent were males.
- Shift workers who work nights or long, irregular hours. Twenty-five million Americans are rotating-shift workers, and 20-30 percent of them report having a sleep-related driving mishap within the prior year.
- Commercial drivers, especially truck drivers. They drive a higher numbers of miles per year, and many must drive at night. Studies find that driver fatigue is associated with 30 to 40 percent of all heavy truck crashes.
- People with untreated sleep disorders. Untreated chronic insomnia, sleep apnea, and narcolepsy can lead to excessive daytime sleepiness that can be fatal. Sleep-related problems affect 50-70 million Americans.

Be a friend to yourself—drive carefully!

About the Author

Dr. Sana Johnson-Quijada is a practicing board certified psychiatrist, a lover of books, a mom, a wife, and a huge fan of Starbucks (as well as local California coffee houses like Maui Wowi Paradise Coffee or Cafe Bravo.)

She is in private practice, specializing in outpatient clinics (in person or by tele-psychiatry, a developing area of remote psychiatry services using technology,) and ECT (electroconvulsive therapy).

She never gets tired of talking about becoming a friend to yourself.

To this end, she blogs at http://friendtoyourself.com, where she hears and shares the concerns and perspectives of self-accountable people in the trenches.

Disclaimer

Stories and details included here come from my imagination, and are not reflective of any patients. The characters are fictitious, not based on real people.

The information in this booklet is provided for general education. Nothing I write is meant to engage the reader in a doctor-patient relationship, nor should it be relied upon as a substitute for professional medical care. Consult your own physician for medical evaluation and treatment.

The purpose of this book is also not to be an academic piece full of footnotes and references. I chose to go with the option of providing material that is readable for the public from any world corner. If you would like to read deeper into these subjects, there is so much more readily available in academic and scientific venues.

Again, thank you for reading.